Live Longer,

FEEL BETTER, AND

Look Great Naked!

Finally, a simple, step-by-step road map to help you weed through all the conflicting and confusing information so you can focus only on what is necessary to look and feel better than you ever thought possible.

RUSS YEAGER

ISBN: 1500765562
ISBN 13: 9781500765569
Library of Congress Control Number: 2014914359
CreateSpace Independent Publishing Platform
North Charleston, South Carolina

This book is dedicated to my amazing clients (past and present); my team of Fitness Coaches, who inspire me every day with their passion, desire, and hard work; and, most of all, to my beautiful wife, Emily, who inspires me not only as an example of health and fitness but as a beautiful and loving person, inside and out.

CONTENTS

Introduction · ix

Chapter 1 How Fast Can I Lose Weight? · · · · · · · · · · · · · · 1
"How can I lose weight in two weeks before _____
(my big vacation, family reunion, etc.)?" · · · · · · · · · · · · · · · 3
"How many pounds can I expect to lose per week?" · · · · · · 3
"What's the best way to lose my belly fat?" · · · · · · · · · · · · 4

Chapter 2 Which Are Better: Free Weights or Machines? · · · 9
"Which equipment do I need to work out?" · · · · · · · · · · · 10
"What are the best exercises?" · 11

Chapter 3 When Is the Best Time to Work Out? · · · · · · · · ·15
"Should I do cardio or weights first?" · · · · · · · · · · · · · · · · 18
"Can I work out two days in a row?" · · · · · · · · · · · · · · · · · 19

Chapter 4 Won't Lifting Weights Make Me Big and Bulky? · · 23
"I feel like my legs and butt get big when
I work out." · 24
"I want to stick to high reps so I don't bulk up." · · · · · · · · 25

Chapter 5 What Do You Think about the _____
Workout? · 29
"Russ, what do you think about CrossFit?" · · · · · · · · · · · · 29
"What about TRX training?" · 31
"Is running bad for your knees?" · · · · · · · · · · · · · · · · · · · 31

Chapter 6　What Is the Best Type of Cardio? · · · · · · · · · · · · 37

High-intensity cardio specifics: · 40

"Did you use this type of cardio to become

lean for your bodybuilding contests?" · · · · · · · · · · · · · · · · 41

Beyond lean high-intensity weekly schedule: · · · · · · · · · · · 42

Chapter 7　What Do You Think about the _____ Diet? · · · · 47

"Should I be following the paleo diet?" · · · · · · · · · · · · · · · 48

"How do I stop the vicious yo-yo diet cycle?" · · · · · · · · · · 50

"How much fruit should I be eating? Should I be

eating fruits at all because of all that sugar?" · · · · · · · · · · · 54

Russ's secret weapon alert: · 55

"How the heck am I supposed to really eat that

many fruits and vegetables *every day*?" · · · · · · · · · · · · · · 56

Chapter 8　Should I Eat Before or After My Workout? · · · · · · ·61

"What if I work out first thing in the morning,

and I'm not hungry?" · 62

"How long before or after my workout should

I eat?" · 62

"What about working out on an empty stomach first

thing in the morning? I heard that this is the best way

to do cardio for fat burning." · 63

"I heard that it's best not to eat after 6:00 p.m. if you

want to lose weight. Is this true?" · · · · · · · · · · · · · · · · · · · 64

"What about alcohol, Russ? I love to have my red wine,

and I don't think I can give it up." · · · · · · · · · · · · · · · · · · · 65

"But I heard red wine has resveratrol and is good

for my heart." · 66

"Can I save up my one or two drinks a night and have

them all in one night?" · 67

Chapter 9   Which Supplements Do I Need to Take? · · · · · · 71

"What do you think of protein shakes and bars?" · · · · · · 73

"I take a multivitamin every day. Won't that cover
all of my bases?" · 74

Bonus Chapter: Motivation, the Mental Edge,
and Getting It Done! · 81

You must have a strong "why" · 82

Motivation · 83

Surround yourself with a positive support system · · · · · · · 84

Never listen to the opinions of negative people! · · · · · · · · 85

Have a deadline · 86

Planning and preparation · 86

Keep a training and nutrition journal · · · · · · · · · · · · · · · · · · 87

Be in control of the situation and not the other
way around · 88

Don't make excuses · 89

Treat each workout as if it were an appointment
with your boss · 90

Use the power of music to fuel your workouts · · · · · · · · · · 91

Keep your eye on the prize · 92

Conclusion and the Ultimate Fat Flush Program · · · · · · · · · · 93

INTRODUCTION

Hello. My name is Russ Yeager. I am a physique transformation specialist and am focused on solving unwanted and frustrating problems, such as weight gain and loss of energy, for women and men over thirty-five.

How did I become a physique transformation expert? I began by transforming myself, as you will read in my story. Then I began getting requests from men and women to help them make their own transformations.

I see the pain in the eyes of so many women and men over thirty-five and hear the frustration in their voices—especially as they get older…as they try to lose weight and get healthier and discover that it's just not as easy as it used to be.

Although I have gotten older (I am about to turn forty at the time of writing this book) and my body does not respond the same way it did in my twenties, I have been able to consistently stay lean, healthy, and full of energy. I've also come to realize that I'm even better at teaching others than I am at teaching myself. That's where my passion really lies—in teaching and helping other people. I can't possibly help all the people in the world who need to lose weight permanently and increase their energy. However, I do have some tools available to help you lose weight quickly and permanently and increase your energy level—even within a matter of a few weeks. Whether you choose to continue down that path or not, I promise you that what you're going to discover in this book will absolutely help you get results.

Ever since I first started lifting weights in high school because my coaches told me to, I have liked the result: muscles! I began learning as much as I could about working out, health, fitness, and nutrition. I obtained a business and accounting degree, because everyone told me that I needed to get a "real" job. In college, I dedicated my electives and all my spare time to learning about the body, nutrition, and working out. I learned a lot and totally transformed my body in the process. I even won an international physique transformation contest in my twenties. However, as I started to get a little older, I noticed that it was getting harder to stay in shape; neither could I eat as much as I once could. That's when I began thinking more about my long-term health and vitality.

Quite frankly, some of the things I was doing to look "lean and mean" were not very healthy, and I often felt exhausted. While I never used the likes of anabolic steroids, I realized that the processed foods, supplements, and overtraining that I used to look good weren't making me any healthier.

This trend continued into my thirties. I felt like I was always struggling with either being healthy or looking good. I would lose weight, gain weight, and repeat this cycle over and over. Sometimes I felt like giving up on a healthy lifestyle altogether! It seemed easier to just eat whatever I wanted and not have to work out, but I knew that it wasn't the path I wanted to take. I decided that I wasn't willing to accept choosing between looking good and being very healthy. I started searching for ways to accomplish both at the same time.

It was in my thirties that I discovered what I now call the Holy Grail of fitness. I finally discovered how I could lose body fat; stay lean and fit; have abundant energy; and enjoy a normal life that didn't revolve around going to the gym and eating dry chicken and bland broccoli all day.

It feels amazing to look and feel better than guys who are ten or even twenty years younger and have the energy and health I need to attend to my career, family, friends, and other important priorities. In my late twenties, I realized that I was getting more questions about nutrition and health than about accounting, and I knew that my calling was to help others transform their lives as well. I have been doing it professionally for over twelve years now, and over the past five, I have created a set of tools and strategies— both physical and mental—to enable men and women over thirty-five to shed body fat quickly, safely, and permanently; and to increase energy levels to match or exceed the energy they had in their twenties.

The goal of this book is to share what I have learned with you, along with helpful additional resources, to help you become the *best you* in the upcoming year!

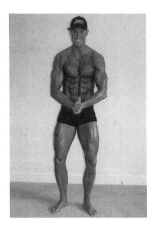 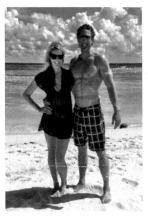

The photo on the left is from 2002, when I won the physique transformation competition. I am very proud of the incredible amount of hard work that I put in, as this event led to the launch of my fitness career and taught me many principles that have helped me and my clients. However, the last few days of extreme carb reduction, dehydration, and electrolyte manipulation (not to mention the ridiculous fake tan)—just to look "perfect" for the pictures—left my exhausted, incredibly irritable, and even in the hospital with a blood clot for five days. I then had to take Coumadin and was unable to work out for three months!

The photo on the right was taken in March of 2014 on the beach in Mexico with my soon-to-be fiancée, Emily. I had followed a strict workout and nutrition plan leading up to the trip, but nothing remotely as extreme as the regimen I had followed in 2002. I can tell you that I felt a heck of a lot better; I even ate pizza and ice cream once a week. I didn't restrict my water or do any crazy nutrient manipulation or anything like that. I look and feel so much healthier, and I haven't experienced any blood clots or other health problems! The picture on the right is a real picture and is representative of the physique I am able to maintain now, year-round, following the principles I share with you in this book. Not too bad for a thirty-nine-year-old guy, if I do say so myself. Just not quite as tan.

CHAPTER 1:

HOW FAST CAN I LOSE WEIGHT?

This is one of the most common questions people ask me: "How fast can I lose (fill in the blank) pounds?" The truth is that dozens and even hundreds of diets can help you lose weight very quickly. The problem is that in most of these short-term diets, the weight loss comes mostly from lean muscle mass and water, rather than fat. After going on one of these typical calorie-restriction diets, you will likely gain the weight back as quickly as you had lost it. Raise your hand if you have been there! I sure have. The big problem is that such diets slow down your metabolism and cannibalize your lean muscle. This phenomenon is even more pronounced when you go on a diet without exercise.

Many experts claim that 80 percent of weight loss boils down to nutrition. While I agree that what you eat is very important, I argue that in order to lose weight (or, more specifically, body fat) safely and permanently, you need the combination of proper nutrition and exercise (more on that later).

The bottom line is that the loss of muscle through diets slows down your metabolism, causing you to gain the weight back. In fact, you are likely to gain even more weight back, since with a lowered metabolism, your body is now burning fewer calories each day.

So what happens next? You go on yet another diet that perpetuates the vicious yo-yo dieting cycle. Not a good place to be! Why? Every time you go on a diet, your metabolism slows down more and more, making it all that more difficult to lose weight permanently. If you have been in this pattern or are in it now, don't lose hope! There is a way to reset your metabolism and keep the weight off.

If you are ready to finally get off the diet merry-go-round and lose fat safely and permanently, read on! You will notice that I keep emphasizing fat weight. It is really important for permanent weight loss. We have been so conditioned to use the number on the scale as the main measurement of success, but weight can be deceiving, nor is it the best measurement of success.

I used to joke with my clients that I could help them lose twenty pounds today. They usually looked at me as though I were crazy, and I'd tell them that I had my chainsaw in the back and that we could take a couple of arms off or maybe a leg. Of course, I was not serious, but I tried to emphasize that it's not necessarily all about losing weight. I also tried to help them understand the importance of not just losing weight, but the importance of losing body fat and maintaining muscle, which will help them have a lean, healthy, and tight physique.

The good news is that you can lose weight, with the majority being body fat, pretty quickly. But the key is to do it properly by following a designed program of strength training, cardiovascular training, and nutrition. We are going to talk a little bit more about how to do that throughout the course of the book.

Through experimenting on myself for twenty years, I have perfected a system that I use with my clients, both in person and remotely, to help them make significant improvements in their physiques, energy levels, and health in only sixty days.

I love the big smiles on my clients' faces when they can't believe how much better they look and feel after only sixty days. However, what I love more is being able to teach them how to maintain their new, healthy body and lifestyle, all without feeling deprived or left out of life.

"HOW CAN I LOSE WEIGHT IN TWO WEEKS BEFORE _____ (MY BIG VACATION, FAMILY REUNION, ETC.)?"

Again, permanent fat loss requires a lifelong commitment to health and fitness. However, it is possible to lose fat and to tone your body very quickly and permanently. The key to doing this is to perform a properly designed program of strength training, cardiovascular training, nutrition, and whole food supplementation, and to do it intensively. This is the secret to losing weight quickly and keeping it off.

I have said many times that the three most important words for success in any fitness plan are *consistency, intensity, and accountability.* Success truly is 80 percent behavior. While this is the cold, hard truth, don't worry. I do have a few tricks and tips that I'll be sharing with you to help make the process more effective and enjoyable.

"HOW MANY POUNDS CAN I EXPECT TO LOSE PER WEEK?"

Again, this is one of the most common questions people ask me. Remember that it's not necessarily all about weight loss and that traditional starvation diets lead to loss of lean muscle mass. As you do it the right way, you will add lean muscle and lose body fat so you may not lose as much scale weight as you would on a traditional starvation diet. But remember that you are going to look better, be healthier, and, most importantly, you're going to be able to keep off the weight permanently.

Common theory says that it's safe to lose one to two pounds a week. This guideline, while helpful for most people, can vary based on age, current weight, gender, and metabolism. Some people can lose weight very quickly, while others lose weight slowly.

However, it is important not to compare yourself to others. Doing so is a recipe for frustration and questioning yourself or your plan. Be concerned only with being the best version of *you* that you can possibly be. Find a program that works for you. Follow it consistently with passion, intensity, and dedication. You will get results.

"WHAT'S THE BEST WAY TO LOSE MY BELLY FAT?"

I'm sure you have seen people at the gym doing hundreds, even thousands of crunches, sit-ups, and ab machine exercises. Yet they never make any progress in their midsection. Maybe that person is you! Heck, we want to believe so badly that we can spot reduce belly fat that we are willing to wear vibrating belts and even rub fat-loss cream on our stomachs. Yes, I admit, I did try the ab cream at one point. Even I am not immune to the relentless marketing of unscrupulous companies offering false hope in the battle of belly fat. The truth is that you can do sit-ups and crunches until you are blue in the face; you simply cannot spot reduce fat. The body simply doesn't work that way.

The process of losing body fat involves the entire body; you cannot choose where to lose the fat. For men, fat usually comes off the arms first, then legs, and finally from the love handles. For women, it typically progresses from arms and chest, midsection, then finally the hips and thighs. I know this is not what you want to hear, and it's not fair. But it's just the way it works. The good news is that once you begin and maintain a proper exercise, nutrition, and supplementation program, *as long as you keep going and don't quit – the fat will come off.*

While we're on the subject of belly fat, it's important to know that the abdomen is one of the most dangerous areas to carry fat, as it carries many health risks. Excessive belly fat significantly increases the risk of cardiovascular disease and many forms of cancer. Since overweight men tend to carry more weight in the belly than overweight women, they have higher rates of heart disease than women, although this can be very dangerous for women as well. So getting the belly fat off is not only important so that you don't have a beer belly and you can feel confident in your clothes or at the beach but also for your health.

Let me reemphasize that you can't spot reduce body fat. You have to follow a properly designed plan. Let the fat come off where it starts—usually your arms—and then keep going. Eventually it will come off your stomach and other stubborn areas as well.

NOTES/ACTION STEPS

CHAPTER 2:

WHICH ARE BETTER: FREE WEIGHTS OR MACHINES?

This is another question that people ask me all the time, and the answer is that it really depends. Both can play a role. I love free weights, because they work the main muscle groups; they require you to stabilize by working the small stabilizer muscles; and they help improve core strength better than machines.

For example, barbell squats involve your core strength more than using a leg press machine does. The benefits of improving core strength and using the stabilizer muscles are, in addition to improved muscle tone and metabolism, a stronger, fitter, and more functional body. You will have an easier time with everyday tasks, become a better athlete, and experience fewer injuries when you are functionally strong.

However, machines do play an important role. The main benefit of machines is that they can be safer. Without a spotter or a personal trainer to watch your form, the use of free weights can get you into trouble and cause serious injury. So machines are a great way to get the great results without the risk of free weights. I think the best approach is first to learn how to work out with free weights under proper supervision and then to combine free weights and machines appropriately.

"WHICH EQUIPMENT DO I NEED TO WORK OUT?"

Walking into the gym can be completely overwhelming—there are so many pieces of equipment! Which do you need to use? The good news is that a great workout doesn't require using a lot of equipment. Some good, old-fashioned barbells and dumbbells are about all that you need. You can also perform many exercises simply with your own body weight.

There have been many times when I am traveling, and have had to stay in very small towns where there are no gyms close by and definitely not a hotel gym. No problem! A few laps around the hotel, some air squats, lunges, jumping jacks, push-ups, and a few burpees and you have a complete, full-body resistance and cardiovascular workout. There are really no excuses for not working out!

While machines do serve a purpose, and while fancy high tech treadmills, elliptical machines, bikes, and stair climbers are nice, there is nothing that stops you from putting on a pair of running shoes, going outside, and hitting the pavement. The truth is that it's usually not the equipment or a lack of knowledge about equipment that prevents us from achieving great results. It's more of a matter of simply taking the time to do the exercises that we set out to do. Finding a knowledgeable buddy—or, even better, hiring a professional trainer—is one of the best ways to learn how to exercise properly. You not only get the best results but also learn how to work out without hurting yourself. If you're hurt, you can't work out at all, and your progress will stop altogether.

"WHAT ARE THE BEST EXERCISES?"

Again, there isn't one clear answer to this question, because your exercise regimen depends on your own personal goals. If your goals are to improve general health and fitness, it's important to perform a variety of exercises that work the major muscle groups. Doing so will help you obtain a well-balanced physique, overall strength, flexibility, and coordination.

I like to focus on performing compound exercises that work the big muscle groups. They help you get the most bang for your buck, so to speak. Some of these compound exercises include squats, barbell bench presses, overhead presses, leg presses, and deadlifts. These exercises can be performed with barbells, dumbbells, TRX, jungle gyms, or your own body weight— the options are endless.

If you are an athlete with specific goals, however, the ideal mix of exercises will likely differ from the above scenario. The regimen you follow will depend on your specific sport, as well as your age, sex, health history, etc. For example, a football lineman who needs to gain strength and speed will not require the same exercises that a ballerina will, who needs to gain core strength, stability, and balance.

In summary, an exercise program needs a variety of strength-training exercises that work all the major muscle groups, cardiovascular training to work your heart, combined with proper nutrition and supplementation to fuel your body so that you can perform optimally, recover well, have a consistent energy level, and maintain optimal health.

NOTES/ACTION STEPS

CHAPTER 3:

WHEN IS THE BEST TIME
TO WORK OUT?

Another common question: Should I work out in the morning, afternoon, or evening?

My answer: the best time to work out is when you'll do it! That's the truth. More important than the time of day, specific exercises, or whether to use free weights or machines is actually doing it and doing it consistently.

Let's imagine two people: we'll call them Person A and Person B. I can give Person A my most disciplined, effective, and complicated workout, in addition to a nutrition and supplementation plan that targets elite athletes. To Person B, I can give a very basic workout routine and nutrition program. If Person B is more consistent and disciplined than Person A, she will likely achieve better results. That's right: consistency trumps the program every time.

Many fitness equipment advertisers would like you to believe that they hold the secret device or workout plan that will let you lose all the weight you want, get in the best shape of your life, and feel amazing with little or no effort. Sorry, but this is just not the case.

Some personal trainers and fitness professionals want you to think that fitness is so complicated that you could never work out on your own and that they have the special program you need. Again, not true.

Why would I say this as a fitness professional? Am I not hurting my business? I don't think so. I honestly believe that hiring a great fitness professional is one of the best health investments you can make. However, the biggest value that fitness coaches and personal trainers provide is to coach, motivate, and push you to levels that you can't achieve on your own. This sense of accountability is much more valuable than the specific plan that they provide. I'm not saying that the specific program isn't important; it is. My point is that consistency is *the* most important element of your exercise program.

You have to do it. You need to have a plan and follow it consistently. Success is 80 percent behavior!

The best time to work out is when you'll actually do it. Now that I have hammered home that point, let's discuss a few advantages of working out in the morning. I prefer to work out early because I know that if I get my workout done in the morning then there is nothing that's going to get in the way of me getting it done for the day.

If I go to work first, it's very possible that I will have a long day, something's going to happen at work, or something else is going to come up that prevents me from working out. It drives me crazy when I miss a workout! Getting it done in the morning eliminates this worry and is also a great way to energize yourself for the rest of the day. Finally, working out the first thing in the morning gives you a sense of accomplishment and pride and will improve your day.

I wish I could say that it gets easier when the alarm clock goes off early and it is still pitch-black outside, but there are still days when all I want to do is hit the snooze button! At least the ringtone on my iPhone is pleasant.

Very rarely, the snooze wins, I sleep in, and I miss my workout. I usually feel disappointed, and my day just doesn't seem to go as well as if I had just gotten my butt up and done what I was supposed to do. However, I have *never* once finished my workout and said, "Boy do I regret that workout." On the contrary, I feel freaking awesome every single time!

After a hard morning workout, I always say to myself, "The hardest part of my day is done. Everything else is going to be a piece of cake!"

If working out in the morning is impossible for you, don't fret. You can work out during lunch, after work, or later in the evening.

I have a client named Eric, whom I work with as a consultant. He works out at 10:00 p.m. or 11:00 p.m., the time of the day that works for him. He's been consistent in working out and has achieved great results. As a side note, Eric had suffered painful rheumatoid arthritis his whole life, had barely ever set foot in a gym, and was a smoker. After only a few short months of consistently following a basic workout, nutrition, and supplementation program, Eric's pain has diminished significantly. He has lost weight, is stronger, feels great, and is no longer a smoker!

Results achieved by real people, like Eric, keep me motivated to wake up early and give my all every single day.

While I have stated my case for morning workouts, any time of day can work. The main thing is a consistent schedule. That's right. You need to schedule your workout into your day and treat it just as you would any business meeting. I advise people to treat their workout time as though it were a meeting with their boss or their most important client. Think about it. You have one body. Isn't taking care of it at least as important as your job, boss, or client?

"SHOULD I DO CARDIO OR WEIGHTS FIRST?"

The main thing is that you just freaking do it! Don't get too caught up in worrying about the order. The order and timing is far less important than the consistency and intensity. However, if you have the flexibility in your schedule and really want to get specific, then you could do your cardiovascular workout and your weight-training workouts separately.

For example, if you do your weight training in the morning, wait until the afternoon or evening to do cardio. The reasoning for this is that strength training and cardio have two very different goals. The goal of strength training is to build muscle and increase strength, which is why you need proper nutrients immediately after the workout. The main goal of the cardio workout is to burn body fat. Combining the two activities in a single session will therefore not give the best results.

How many of us have the time to work out once a day, much less twice? So, that tip is applicable only to those who are at the level of elite athletes and have the time to train extensively. Such workouts are commonly referred to as "two-a-days."

If you combine weight training and cardio, I recommend doing weight training before the cardio, as lifting heavier weights requires greater exertion. As long as you are eating properly, you will primarily consume glycogen as fuel during weight-training workouts, which leaves body fat to be burned during cardio.

You can also do cardio before strength training. I've done this and have gotten good results. Having used myself as a guinea pig to test everything, I have found certain strategies more effective than others. However, I'll repeat once again that *the most important factors in working out are consistency and intensity.* You need to work out hard and consistently to create positive change.

Another question people often ask me is the subject of frequent debate...

"CAN I WORK OUT TWO DAYS IN A ROW?"

That's a great question, and the answer is *yes,* absolutely!

This question comes up because people understand the body's need to recover after a workout, especially strength training. But it's easy to set up split routines, e.g. working your upper body one day and your lower body the next, or perhaps weights one day and cardiovascular or functional training the next.

Often, my clients will travel and be away from the gym on Thursday and Friday, while their workout plan calls for a Monday-Wednesday-Friday routine. They can adjust their workout schedule to Monday-Tuesday-Wednesday routine in such a case. Traveling is not a problem as long as your workout schedule allows different parts of the body to rest. In addition, the total amount of work and load placed on each muscle group and your body overall on a weekly basis is more important than the days of the week each type of workout is performed.

Diet, rest, and stress levels all affect the speed of recovery.

NOTES/ACTION STEPS

CHAPTER 4:

WON'T LIFTING WEIGHTS MAKE ME BIG AND BULKY?

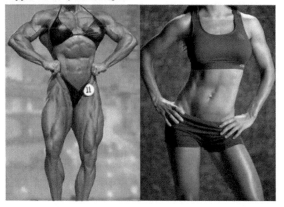

What women think will happen if they lift weights... What actually happens...

What Women Think They'll Look Like   What Will Actually Happen!
If They Lift Heavy Weights

This is a question I get, mostly from women.

One of the biggest misconceptions about strength training is that it will make women big and bulky. This simply is *not true!* Women lack the testosterone levels of men, making it almost impossible for them to build enough muscle to become big and bulky. Actually, strength-training exercises are very important for women, because they speed up metabolism and help burn body fat.

In fact, every pound of lean muscle burns an extra twenty to forty calories per day. This is one of the secrets of strength training and explains why weights help you become lean and stay that way. This is *so* important. Please do not ignore this! Read it again, and make sure that it sinks in.

Think about it. You are actually creating a situation where you are burning excess calories even when you are not doing anything. I like to compare this to the power of investing your money and having it work for you, even though you are not physically doing anything. This is a very powerful concept!

I can guarantee that the women you see who are very fit, tight, and toned are using strength training in their fitness programs. The truth is that women who feel big and bulky don't have excess muscle; it's fat that's covering up their muscle. Following a properly designed program of strength training, cardio, and nutrition will take off the body fat, and will reveal, underneath, lean, smooth, and beautiful muscle.

I tell all my female clients that if they start getting too muscular, we'll scale back the strength training. In over fourteen years, it hasn't happened yet.

"I FEEL LIKE MY LEGS AND BUTT GET BIG WHEN I WORK OUT."

If you feel this way, you are building some lean muscle, but body fat is making you look big and bulky. Further reducing body fat will make you love strength training, because it's going to make your hips, thighs, and butt toned, fit, and sexy!

"I WANT TO STICK TO HIGH REPS SO I DON'T BULK UP."

Again, this is something I hear mostly from my female clients. I have to sit them down and honestly tell them the importance of lifting through a variety of low, medium, and high repetition ranges. I would be doing a disservice to my clients by making them only do high repetitions, when I know that the results that they are seeking require working through all the ranges.

Understanding how the body works and the differences in hormone levels between men and women will help you understand that you won't build too much muscle.

Heck, I'm a man, and I feel like I have to fight tooth and nail for every pound of muscle that I gain.

If you are still having a hard time with this concept then you need to go back and look at the picture at the beginning of this chapter again!

If you don't believe me, ask the next woman you see with a lean and toned figure (not big or bulky) about her workouts. I'll bet you a protein shake that she lifts weights. Sure, there is always the nineteen-year-old or the genetic freak who will look great without doing anything, but she's the exception. The rest of us, men and women alike, need to lift hard and heavy to produce the most fit, most beautiful, and sexiest versions of ourselves.

As we discussed in the previous chapter, focusing on compound exercises that recruit the large muscle groups will create the biggest metabolism boost and thus fat-burning effect. So, learn proper form and then go get your squat on!

In summary, performing compound strength-training exercises at the right intensity is one of the single most effective strategies for increasing your metabolism; losing body fat permanently; and staying fit, beautiful, and lean.

NOTES/ACTION STEPS

CHAPTER 5:

WHAT DO YOU THINK ABOUT THE _____ WORKOUT?

People often ask me what I think about a particular type of workout. Probably the most common question is:

"RUSS, WHAT DO YOU THINK ABOUT CROSSFIT?"

CrossFit has become extremely popular very quickly, and CrossFit gyms (or boxes, as they are sometimes referred to) are popping up everywhere.

My answer concerning Crossfit and any other type of fitness program consists of the following advice:

1) Find a workout program that makes sense to you and that you are going to be able to follow consistently with belief and passion. Your belief and how comfortable and confident you are about a program is going to play a big role in your consistency.

2) Before beginning the program, it's important to make sure that the workout is both safe and effective and that it will be a good fit to help you reach your goals.

3) Do the instructors seem knowledgeable? Do they make sense? Do they have credibility and credentials?

Have they helped other clients with goals and challenges similar to yours? Do they stand behind their services and offer a money-back guarantee?

4) It is important to visit the gym or the personal training environment where you'll be working out. Ask them if they are willing to let you try a free workout before you make a decision. They should be willing to do this for you. Make sure that it is the best fit for you and that you feel great about the environment and the people.

5) Trust your instincts. Do some research, have a conversation, talk to current and past clients of the person supplying your workout program. Whether it's a personal trainer, a group instructor, or a fitness DVD creator, you want to make sure that the person knows what they are doing. Find someone who is competent and inspires confidence.

Trust your instincts in these situations. If you don't feel comfortable, don't feel pressured. Ask many questions. It is an encouraging sign when a trainer asks a lot of questions. Because everyone is different, it's important that a professional knows a lot about your goals, needs, existing health issues, or anything else that may affect your program. The trainer will then be able to design a program that is both effective and safe for you.

One word of caution about information overload. It is easy to fall into the trap of feeling that you need to get all the information before getting started. This leads to procrastination, and you will not improve if you aren't working out! When you find a plan that you feel good about, take action and start right away! Thinking about it doesn't change your body or your life. Making decisions and taking action do!

"WHAT ABOUT TRX TRAINING?"

TRX is another big buzz-word these days and it has also become very popular. Many fitness programs have been created that focus on TRX training. TRX is a very popular brand of suspension training.

Suspension training involves two handles attached to a stable surface, such as pull-up bars, with strong straps that allows you to do a variety of exercises using your own body weight. There are several different brands, but TRX is the most popular (and most expensive).

I prefer to use the Jungle Gym brand of suspension training in my studios, but both are very good.

Suspension training can be a very effective form of exercise. However, the equipment that you use matters less than the type of movements you're performing, the overall program you are following, and the intensity level of your workouts.

"IS RUNNING BAD FOR YOUR KNEES?"

People also ask me a lot of questions about running. There is no doubt that good, old-fashioned running has its advantages. It's tough to do, but running burns a lot of calories and can really get us into shape quickly. Plus, you don't need any equipment, even a treadmill. Just get good running shoes, go outside, hit the pavement and you're on your way.

Running does put a lot of pressure on your knees and joints, so it's important to be smart and pay attention to your body. If you have bad knees and they feel worse after running, it may not be the best activity for you.

Often, simple measures, such as getting a professional shoe-fitting and running on softer surfaces, such as the beach or wooded trails, can help alleviate pain associated with running on concrete or in old or ill-fitting shoes.

Since I'm a big guy (6'6," 225 lbs.), running puts a lot of stress on my body. I like to run, and I know that it is great exercise. But because my body is not ideally suited for running, I limit my runs to once or twice per week. Getting fitted for shoes by a professional made a world of difference in both my performance and how my body feels when I run.

I recently started working with a podiatrist who specializes in improving athletic performance and reducing pain. He has worked with collegiate and professional athletes as well as the Navy Seals. His philosophy is that no one is created totally symmetrical, and that virtually all of us have one leg that is longer than the other.

He believes that over time this imbalance not only prevents us from performing optimally in athletics, but also contributes to the majority of arthritis pain we typically associate with aging or "overuse" syndrome.

This doctor creates custom orthotics designed to correct these imbalances, which reduces joint stress and pain and allows you to perform at a higher level. He explains it as "putting eye glasses on a sharp shooter."

I have been using the orthotics created for me for a few months and can tell a reduction in the amount of pain in my left hip. I have suffered from hip pain for about 7 years and finally found out I have very little cartilage in my left hip. I feel like the orthotics are making a positive difference, and have started recommending that some of my clients take a look at this as an option for pain relief and improvement in athletic performance.

I know this section is about running, but the biggest difference I have noticed since I started using custom orthotics is an improvement in my squats. My feet naturally turn in or pronate. When squatting, the weight on my back causes even more pronation of my feet and my knees start to "buckle" when the weight gets heavy.

With my orthotics, as well as some shoes selected to help create a more favorable starting position for my feet, my squats feel much more stable, my knees don't buckle, and I can even lift more weight. This is a new discovery for me and I definitely don't claim to be an expert or that this is a "cure all" solution for everyone. I just like to share with others anything that has helped me along my fitness and health journey. As with anything, not all podiatrist and not all orthotics are created equal so if you decide to give them a try I recommend doing your research, and then evaluating your own personal results.

Another strategy I have used consistently for years is getting sports massages on a regular basis. I believe that regular sports massages are one of the best things you can do to reduce aches and pains associated with running and other physical activities.

Again, do your research and try different massage therapists as not all are created equal. There are some very talented therapists out there that understand the body and specialize in pain relief and corrective therapy. Staying pain free through massage therapy not only makes life more enjoyable, but can help improve strength, endurance, flexibility, and overall athletic performance.

Even though there are things you can do to reduce pain and make running more tolerable, running may not be for everyone. A good rule of thumb is that if something causes you pain either find a way to perform that activity differently so the pain disappears, or just quit doing it all together!

If you have special situations where your body has been hurt and your knees or hips are injured more by running then there's a lot of other things you can do to get the same cardiovascular benefit without the pounding that running puts on your knees. A few examples include swimming, elliptical machines, or biking (either stationary, street, or mountain bike).

My favorite cardio activity is the gauntlet. I like to call it "big steps." You may have seen the big steps at the gym that go around in a circle. You simply step up and down, but if you don't keep up, you fall off the back. How's that for motivation? I like it, because I can crank up my iPod, listen to my favorite music or book, and get an awesome cardio workout with no real impact on my knees or joints.

NOTES/ACTION STEPS

CHAPTER 6:

WHAT IS THE BEST TYPE OF CARDIO?

Cardiovascular exercise should be part of any good fitness program. Fat burning is one of the main benefits of cardiovascular training. Other benefits of cardio exercise include reduced blood pressure, overall better heart health, improved concentration and mood, better recoverability, and increased energy.

Cardiovascular exercise can be performed in many different ways and at various levels of intensity, all with their own benefits. There is an ongoing debate over high-intensity cardio and low-intensity cardio. Both types of cardio can be effective and have their place, and both are supported by scientific studies. What I am going to share is based on my personal experience and the experience of my clients.

I believe that high-intensity cardio cannot be beaten for becoming really lean quickly. High-intensity interval training can be completed in as few as sixteen to twenty minutes. Achieving the same results from low-intensity cardio would require three or four times that.

People often cannot believe that many of my cardio sessions last just sixteen to twenty minutes. However, when they see me perform cardio, in person or on my Complete Physique Training DVD, they understand that this type of cardio is very intense. In fact, it can even be brutally difficult. However, I don't mind the intensity, because I know how extremely effective it is at burning fat. I have also found short, intense cardio sessions to have a minimal negative impact on muscle building efforts, as long as my nutrition is in order.

The reason that intense cardio is so effective is because it increases your metabolic rate much more than moderate- or low-intensity cardio does. When your metabolism is cranked up through intense cardiovascular exercise, it will continue to soar for hours after your cardio session is over, so you will continue to burn calories at an accelerated rate.

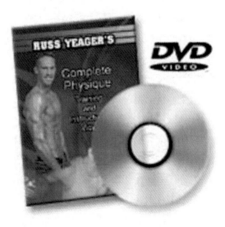

My Complete Physique Training DVD demonstrates the type of cardio and weight training intensity necessary to turn your body into a fat-burning furnace. You can get a copy at special discounted price by visiting: www.yourcompletephysique.com.

If you think about it, intense cardio workouts are a huge return on a relatively small investment. If you could achieve such returns in business, the decision to make the investment would be a no brainer, so why should it be any different with your body?

Even if your main goal is increased lean muscle mass, cardio should be a regular part of your training program. In addition to the health benefits, performing intense cardiovascular exercise can actually help you achieve your muscle-building goals. Intense cardio improves blood flow to the muscles and increases the volume of blood contained in the blood vessels and veins, creating a cell-volumizing effect. This means that your muscles literally expand similar to what occurs during strength training, although not to the same extent.

Intense cardio also increases your metabolism, allowing you to eat more muscle-building calories without adding unwanted body fat. Finally, intense cardio also provides an anabolic response and protects against muscle breakdown, which can occur with longer cardio sessions. Remember that lean muscle drives your metabolism and keeps you lean. Let me reiterate to my female audience that lean muscle does *not* mean that you will be big and bulky! Please remember that and trust me on this. My goal is to help you do things differently than the average person who believes certain things, so that you can get different results than the average person.

When comparing high-intensity and low-intensity cardio, think of the difference between a sprinter's body and a marathon runner's body. We all know that the sprinter is very lean and has visible muscle while the marathon runner is softer and carries very little muscle.

Intense cardio exercise takes some getting used to and also requires some mental and physical toughness. It is extremely demanding, but ever since I have been doing cardio this way I can't imagine doing it any other way. Time is one of the most valuable resources we have, and intense, short-duration cardio saves you lots of it. I spend sixteen to twenty minutes while others spend up to an hour or more on the treadmill or bike without achieving the results they are after.

HIGH-INTENSITY CARDIO SPECIFICS:

High-intensity cardio is often referred to as HIIT (high-intensity interval training) cardio. While HIIT can take on a number of forms, the main idea is to perform cardio for a specified length of time, and within that duration to work at various intensity intervals. For example, you can perform twenty minutes of cardio and alternate between high-intensity and recovery intervals of one minute. You would thus perform ten high-intensity intervals during the twenty-minute session. Another way to perform high-intensity cardio is to steadily increase the intensity over two or three minutes until you reach a peak intensity level, then reduce the intensity a few notches and work back up so that you hit several peaks during your cardio session. Yet another way to perform high-intensity cardio is to simply go as hard as you possibly can for sixteen, twenty, or thirty minutes.

Any of these variations will work as long as you are truly pushing yourself. A good way to ensure you continually raise your cardio standards, and also add a competitive aspect is to turn your cardio into a game by tracking your calories and distance on the cardio equipment. The goal is to beat your previous performance every cardio session. If you strive to do this, you are forced to produce some very intense cardio sessions whether you always reach your goal or not. It takes time to build up your level of intensity, so start off slow and be patient.

I suggest performing cardio two to four times per week for general health. If your goal is to lose as much fat as possible, or to get ready for a beach trip or a reunion, I recommend performing cardio more often—up to seven days a week, and even twice a day, depending on how much fat you wish to lose and how much time you have.

I normally perform my intense cardio sessions using a stair stepper, a step mill, or a recumbent bike (this is the stationary bike where you are sitting down and slightly leaning back). I simply prefer these three pieces of equipment, but don't feel limited to the bike, the stair stepper, or even staying inside. Running stadiums is an outstanding way to skyrocket your heart rate and metabolism. You can apply intense interval training to almost any activity, including running, biking, swimming, or jumping rope. Other great cardio options include playing full-court basketball, mountain biking, and high-intensity aerobic or spinning classes. Although these forms of exercise will probably take more time than twenty minutes and may not be quite as intense, they are very effective at burning fat, provided that you push yourself.

"DID YOU USE THIS TYPE OF CARDIO TO BECOME LEAN FOR YOUR BODYBUILDING CONTESTS?"

Yes, I sure did. For those who are interested in losing a lot of fat quickly, here is the exact cardio plan that I shared in an article I wrote for *Natural Muscle and Fitness* Magazine. It is intense and will help you burn a lot of fat. However, you must also eat properly in order to see significant changes in your physique. Otherwise, you risk overeating and negating the fat-burning effects of your workout. It is *very tough* to out-exercise a bad diet. After one holiday season of overindulging in delicious but not so healthy foods, and trying to make up for it by performing cardio every day, I concluded that it is actually *impossible* to out-exercise a bad diet; although it sure is fun to try!

BEYOND LEAN HIGH-INTENSITY WEEKLY SCHEDULE:

Day of Week	Cardio Equipment	Duration	Format
Sunday	Rest day	Rest day	Rest day
Monday	Stair stepper (In the evening after weight training in the morning)	20 minutes	Hill setting
Tuesday	Recumbent bike (In the evening after weight training in the morning)	16 minutes	Manual setting (alternate between one-minute all-out sprint and one-minute moderate-intensity intervals)
Wednesday	Step mill (gauntlet)—In the morning (no weight training)	30 minutes	Rolling hills setting at moderate to high intensity during entire session
Thursday	Recumbent bike (In the evening after weight training in the morning)	16 minutes	Manual setting (alternate between one-minute all-out sprint and one-minute moderate-intensity intervals)
Friday	Stair stepper (In the evening after weight training in the morning)	20 minutes	Hill setting
Saturday	Step mill (gauntlet)—In the morning (no weight training)	30 minutes	Rolling hills setting at moderate to high intensity during entire session

I work up to this schedule from my two to three sessions per week off-season cardio schedule by adding one cardio session per week. If needed, I will add an additional intense cardio session per week to the schedule above. I will add a seventh session on Sunday and then begin performing double cardio sessions (one at lunch and one in the evening) on the other days—up to fourteen sessions per week, or until I reach my body-fat percentage goal.

Please keep in mind that when performing this many cardio sessions per week I was preparing for a bodybuilding competition in which you must be extremely lean. While everyone is different, if you are consistently performing intense cardio 5-7 days per week, following a consistent nutrition plan with controlled calorie intake, and performing intense strength training, you should be able to achieve a "beach-ready" physique with visible abdominal muscles.

Of course, the more body fat you start with the longer it will take to get into shape. The key is to track if you are making progress. If you are then keep doing what you are doing. If not, then give it another few weeks and if you are still not making progress then it is time to reassess and make some adjustments.

NOTES/ACTION STEPS

CHAPTER 7:

WHAT DO YOU THINK ABOUT THE _____ DIET?

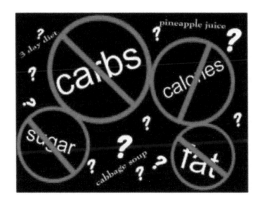

South Beach, Atkins, high carb, low carb, vegan, Paleo diet: the list goes on and on.

New diets seem to come out just about every week, and I often receive questions about them. I also hear story after story about someone who followed a particular diet and lost weight but gained it back as soon as he or she stopped following the diet.

The regaining of weight is the main problem with diets, along with the fact that they are so hard to stick to! There is a reason that the first three letters of diet are D-I-E. It's because you feel like you're going to die!

"SHOULD I BE FOLLOWING THE PALEO DIET?"

The paleo diet is one of the diets that has gained a lot of popularity.

This diet is based on the premise that the paleolithic man, or the caveman, ate lots of meat, very few carbohydrates other than fruits and vegetables, and some nuts and seeds. Gluten, dairy, and grains are prohibited from the paleo diet. The idea is to exclude processed foods and to live on fat and protein.

I believe that this is one of the better diets. However, the challenge is to follow it consistently! To avoid eating carbohydrates apart from fruits and vegetables is impractical for many. Also, for an endurance athlete, it can be hard to get the energy required to fuel long workouts.

My experience has been that the paleo diet is not the best for my needs. In fact, no diet is the best solution. Just by knowing that you are on a diet, you are psychologically induced to think of it as a short-term situation. When you stop a short-term diet, you lose your focus, and your results go away.

I like to find an eating program that works for me all the time and teach my clients to do the same. You may have periods during which you follow your nutrition program strictly, perhaps to accomplish a short-term or midrange goal. There may be times when you are a little more relaxed, such as during the holidays. However, the overall structure and foundation of the plan should remain the same. Do not follow a diet that sets you up for short-term results and long-term failure.

Many of us wonder why we gain all the weight back after stopping a diet. Doesn't it make sense that, if you revert to your previous eating habits, you should at least keep the weight off that you had lost? It simply doesn't work that way. Here's the reason: going on a diet typically decreases our caloric intake to a very low level, which leads to weight loss.

If you ingest fewer calories than you burn, you will lose weight. However, it is important to consider the type of weight lost. When on a low-calorie diet, you will typically experience three types of weight reduction:

1) You first lose water weight, especially if you're on a low-carbohydrate diet, because each gram of carbohydrates holds a significant amount of water. As you eliminate carbohydrates from your diet, you also lose water.
2) You will lose some body fat.
3) Very often (and this is the big problem!), you will also lose lean muscle weight.

So, let's consider a woman who weighs 175 pounds and loses thirty pounds in three months. Let's say ten pounds of the lost weight comes from lean muscle, a likely scenario, especially if she is not exercising and her calories are highly restricted. Her basal metabolic rate is now lower than it had been before she started the diet. So when she returns to her normal caloric intake, she gains all the weight back that she lost, and even some additional weight, because her metabolic rate is lower than it had been before. The number on the scale is lower initially, but she has set herself up for even more long-term struggles with her weight.

Once the weight is back on, she goes on another diet again, only to have the weight return. This time, she has lowered her metabolism even more. This is the vicious cycle of yo-yo dieting that many of us have been through.

"HOW DO I STOP THE VICIOUS YO-YO DIET CYCLE?"

What I follow and recommend is to eat in a way that stabilizes your blood sugar level. This takes place mostly with healthy foods but also with less healthy treats that you nevertheless enjoy. This helps you get the necessary nutrients from healthy foods without the sense that you're depriving yourself, which can lead to binging. Believe me; I have been there!

Keeping stable blood sugar is the key, and the three main factors for doing so are:

1) Eating small, frequent meals throughout the day, about once every three hours.
2) Having the proper amount of calories in each meal. This number depends on one's age, metabolism, gender, goals, exercise program, and other factors.

Determining the proper range of calories per meal and per day is something I can help figure out for my clients individually. However, as a starting point, most people's needs will fall somewhere between two hundred and six hundred calories per meal. It may be closer to two hundred for a woman who is not very active and who has a lot of weight to lose, while it may be closer to six hundred for a very active man. The calorie needs may be even higher for an elite athlete.

It is important to break these meals into five or six smaller meals throughout the day. Doing so supplies the body with a consistent flow of nutrients and increases the metabolism, in addition to stabilizing blood sugar levels.

Eating this way takes some getting used to. It is very different from the traditional idea of three square meals a day, or even a single or two daily meals that many Americans eat. You may feel as if you are not eating enough at first, but the good news is that you only have to wait a few more hours to eat again. Be patient with it, and remind yourself of the payoff of a faster metabolism, more consistent energy, and a leaner body for life!

3) Getting the proper macronutrient ratio in each meal. That simply means having the correct proportion of protein, carbohydrate, and fat in each meal. While there is no exact formula, a good starting point is to have about 40 percent of your calories come from carbohydrates (try to focus on most of these carbs being wholesome, unprocessed, low-glycemic carbohydrates. Think veggies!), about 30 percent from lean protein sources, and about 30 percent from fat sources.

That's right; 30 percent of your daily calories should come from fat. This goes against what many of us have heard about fat being bad. Fat is very important for a lot of reasons. Not only is fat a good source of fuel for our bodies, it also plays an important role in hormonal balance and other functions of the body, as well as our overall health.

The key is to eat the healthy types of fat. Healthy fats, such as omega-3 fats, are found in sources, such as fish oil, salmon, and some nuts and seeds. Other healthy fats include olive oil, nut butter, and avocado. Guacamole, used as salad dressing, is delicious and healthy!

On the other hand, excessive unhealthy fat can cause major health problems and weight gain. The fats that we should try to avoid include saturated fats and trans fats. As you read food labels, look out for anything with partially hydrogenated fats. These are genetically modified trans fats and are bad news. They are very bad for us and are mostly found in processed foods.

If you stick to whole foods, you don't have to worry about these fats.

A good rule of thumb when buying food is that the fewer ingredients, the better. If it comes in a box or a bag, and there is a long list of ingredients that you don't recognize or can't even pronounce, you are better off staying away. In contrast, it is hard to go wrong if you stick to the produce section. For example, there is only one ingredient for an apple: apple!

Having the correct balance of macronutrients in each meal is the most difficult part of the equation in the beginning. Once you learn how to do this and get used to it, it becomes second nature and one of your most powerful allies for being able to get lean, stay lean, and have consistent energy levels throughout the day.

Once this nutrition routine becomes a way of life, keeping your weight under control and having the energy you need every day will be much easier. Fortunately, you can make this work with any type of food.

It's true. If you control your calories at each meal, eat every three hours or so consistently, and have the proper amount of macronutrients in each meal, you will lose body fat and stay lean. However, as I learned from my bodybuilding days, being lean does not always equal being healthy. Long-term health depends not only on the quantity of the food we eat but also on its quality.

A great plan is to focus on most of your food coming from wholesome whole foods such as fruits, vegetables, grains and healthy fats. It is ok to incorporate some of the not so healthy but delicious "fun" food that we all like to enjoy as well. In fact, this is one of the keys to enjoying your eating plan and making it something you can do for the rest of your life, as opposed to a diet.

Another benefit of eating this way for a long time is that your body becomes very efficient at processing calories. So, having a cheat or splurge day won't mess up your progress. Your metabolism will keep going and your body will simply expel the unneeded fats and calories.

The key here is first to reach your ideal body type and weight goal before having these splurge or cheat days. Also, make sure that you keep it to a splurge meal or, at most, a splurge day. Stringing together days of overeating will slow down your metabolism, make you feel sluggish, and lead to weight gain.

Be very careful here. Although you may not notice any difference after only a few days of overeating, it can sneak up on you. You might exclaim in surprise, "What the heck? I was just looking great, and now I am fat!" I can speak about this from personal experience.

One of my personal training clients, Chris, and I are always joking about how we work so hard for weeks and months to get our "six pack" abs and then can wipe them out with one big eating day on the weekend!

I have also noticed that of the few times I get sick, it is typically during the holidays when I am eating more unhealthy foods. In Western society, we think of illness being generating externally from germs, but what is going on inside of our bodies is a big determining factor of whether we get sick or not. This is just one more reason to focus on eating mostly healthy food and limiting sugar and processed foods.

One very interesting question people often ask me is:

"HOW MUCH FRUIT SHOULD I BE EATING? SHOULD I BE EATING FRUITS AT ALL BECAUSE OF ALL THAT SUGAR?"

While it is true that fruit contains sugar, your body processes the sugar found in fruit very differently from how it processes sugar in processed foods, such as cereal, candy bars, chips, and more.

Fruit is one of the healthiest foods there is, and is full of phytonutrients, vitamins, minerals, and antioxidants. We need a wide variety of fruits and vegetables in our diet, and it's important to eat them consistently. It is true that sugar from fruits, in excess, can keep you from losing weight and cause a sugar spike. However it's very difficult to overeat fruit.

If I eat an apple, two oranges, and a big bunch of grapes, then I am going to be completely satisfied, and I have only consumed about three hundred calories or so, the equivalent of a very small bowl of cereal or a Pop-Tart. Once you are satisfied after eating fruit, you remain satisfied. With processed foods, however, it's very easy to continue to crave and to ingest a thousand calories or more of processed sugar in one sitting. Talk about a blood sugar disaster!

I have *never once* met anyone who struggled with weight as a result of eating too much fruit. Please! Let's be honest! It ain't the fruit that's making us fat! It's all the other crap we our putting in our bodies, half the time unconsciously, combined with a lack of daily exercise and overall movement. (And, yes, I am from Alabama where *ain't* is a real word when you are trying to make a point!)

So don't be afraid of fruit. Be sure to include a few servings a day into your diet.

Let's also talk about vegetables. Vegetables are the single most nutritious food that we can eat. Vegetables are loaded with antioxidants, phytonutrients, vitamins, minerals, and fiber. Scientific research is discovering more and more benefits of vegetables every year. The news isn't that fruits and vegetables are good for us—it's that they are so good for us that they just may save our lives!

The most recent recommendation is that half of our plate should consist of fruits and vegetables, or the equivalent of seven to thirteen servings of fruits and vegetables a day. Good luck! This can be very challenging to follow, but it's important that we make an effort to get as close as we can.

It is also important that we consume a wide variety of fruits and vegetables, not just ones that we like. I used to eat only green beans and apples. While those are both very healthy, I wasn't getting the full spectrum of the nutrients that are present in the rainbow of colors of fruits and vegetables.

When I was a kid I didn't like any vegetables! In fact, I remember picking the onions out of my mom's chili! I have come a long way and do a better job of eating my vegetables now. Even though a bowl of cereal or big sandwich may provide more instant gratification, knowing the amazing health benefits of vegetables motivates me to eat as many as I can.

Vegetables also offer one more very powerful benefit…

RUSS'S SECRET WEAPON ALERT:

There is one more unique characteristic possessed by vegetables that I have used for myself and my clients as a "secret weapon" to help lose body fat. Vegetables are the one food that we can literally eat as much of as we want. Yep (Alabama, remember?), that's right. You cannot overeat vegetables, so chow down!

The reason for this is that it takes a certain amount of calories just to digest the food that we eat. Vegetables are so nutrient dense that we can eat a tremendous amount of them, and the total calories consumed are still very low. Additionally, the amount of fiber in vegetables is so high that it increases your metabolism and causes your body to work and burn calories to digest the vegetables.

A big bag of broccoli or green beans may only be a hundred calories, but can be very satisfying. Your body requires almost as many calories as are found in the vegetables just to digest them. So the net caloric intake comes to nearly zero. I don't even count vegetable calories in my daily total. When I was competing in natural bodybuilding, I would literally eat pounds of veggies every day and reach sub-5-percent body fat levels. Vegetables are truly the one food that you can eat as much as you want.

Naturally, there are exceptions. Starchy vegetables, like corn, are one exception. It is possible to ingest too many calories by overeating corn. However, with the fibrous vegetables, such as broccoli, cauliflower, green beans, and spinach, there is no limit to the quantity, and they can be quite delicious. Try adding some light seasoning and olive oil. You *do* need to count the calories from olive oil, seasoning, and anything else used in cooking.

Makes, sense Russ, but…

"HOW THE HECK AM I SUPPOSED TO REALLY EAT THAT MANY FRUITS AND VEGETABLES *EVERY DAY?*"

Because it is often difficult to eat enough fruits and vegetables, it is important to look at a few options that can make getting them into your diet easier. One solution is making smoothies or juicing. It can be a great way to get a lot of nutrients quickly and efficiently. There are many great recipes for fruit and vegetable smoothies. Smoothies even taste great too!

The downside of juicing and smoothies is that it does take some time to purchase, clean, organize, and cut the produce to make the juice or smoothie. You also have to be disciplined about following through and actually doing it. It takes time to buy all of the produce and it can get expensive fast. It seems like it takes a tremendous amount of vegetables and fruit to get just a small amount of juice. I always felt like I was throwing away more of the fruits and vegetables than I was juicing because it would go bad before I could get to it. Does this sound familiar at all?

I was lucky enough to find another solution that has worked very well for me and many of my clients for many years now. This solution is called Juice Plus. Juice Plus consists of twenty-eight fruits, vegetables, and berries grown fresh in the field, picked at the peak of vine ripeness, juiced, dried at low temperatures, and put into a convenient capsule or gummy form. Some of the biggest benefits of Juice Plus are convenience and time saved. Anyone can get in the habit of taking a few capsules a day (remember that we need seven to thirteen servings of fruits and vegetables every day, not three or four days a week!). Another great benefit of Juice Plus is the cost savings. Juice Plus costs less than $2.50 a day. Trying to get the equivalent amount of fruits and vegetables in whole food form, or through juicing or smoothies, will cost significantly more.

One important final note on Juice Plus. I believe that it is the most convenient, effective, and economic way to get more fruits and vegetables into our diet. I also believe that everyone on the planet should be adding Juice Plus to their diet, regardless of how many fruits and vegetables he or she eats every day because everyone has a gap either in quantity or variety. Juice Plus does just that, bridges the gap. It is not a replacement for eating fruits and vegetables. It is important that we get adequate amounts of fiber that can only be obtained by eating whole fruits and vegetables.

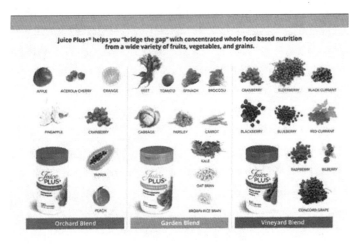

Juice Plus+® helps you "bridge the gap" with concentrated whole food based nutrition from a wide variety of fruits, vegetables, and grains.

For more information on Juice Plus, visit **www.russ.juiceplus.com**.

Can you tell I am passionate about nutrition? Perhaps by the fact that this was the longest chapter in the book so far. I am very passionate about it and have a lot to say because the "eating part" is almost always the hardest part for each of us.

The key is to apply the strategies and resources I provided and always work towards getting better and better. If you mess up and fall down, don't beat yourself up! It's OK! Just get back on it and always strive to improve. We should strive for excellence, not perfection.

Ok, I have worked up an appetite, and it has been three hours since my last meal. I'm going to go refuel with some veggies, lean ground turkey, and almonds. I'll be back to talk about how to time your meals around your workouts.

NOTES/ACTION STEPS

CHAPTER 8:

SHOULD I EAT BEFORE OR AFTER MY WORKOUT?

When is the most important time to eat? How important is the timing of my meals?

While there's no single answer to this question, the most important thing to remember is that our bodies need a consistent supply of good nutrition every day. It is therefore ideal to eat both before and after your workout. The timing, however, depends on your particular goals and needs, as well as when you're working out in the day.

One very powerful nutritional strategy for building muscle and improving recovery is to have a nutritious meal or shake both before your workout and immediately following your workout, then follow this up with another nutritious meal within two hours.

Your body needs most of its energy centered around your workouts. Think about it: most of us have office jobs and expend very little physical energy during most of the day. A workout dramatically increases your body's demand for energy and nutrients. This is especially true of intense workouts (which I recommend to get maximum results). If you can be diligent and take advantage of this unique three-hour window of opportunity, you will have a big jump-start on getting awesome results from your workout and nutrition plan.

These pre- and postworkout meals should have lean protein, complex carbohydrates, and a little bit of healthy fat. You can have a whole meal or a meal replacement shake.

I like to use a meal replacement shake because it is convenient and supplies energy quickly to my body both before and after my workout. The liquid form gets absorbed more quickly than the whole foods and thus provides quick energy and recovery. However, more important than choosing between shakes or meals is getting consistent, quality nutrition before and after your workouts.

"WHAT IF I WORK OUT FIRST THING IN THE MORNING, AND I'M NOT HUNGRY?"

At 5:00 a.m. it may be difficult to get in a full meal. This is where a nutritional shake or a meal replacement shake can be a great solution. I have had a handful of clients who simply could not tolerate eating before their morning workout. This is where you have to be flexible, smart, and willing to listen to your body.

If eating before the morning workout makes you sick, don't eat just to try to get "ideal" nutrition. But be sure to drink some water before and during your workout, and follow it up with a nutritious postworkout meal or shake.

"HOW LONG BEFORE OR AFTER MY WORKOUT SHOULD I EAT?"

Again, there is no single, perfect answer for everyone. It depends on your goals and on how you feel during the workout. For example, I like to have my preworkout shake about thirty to forty-five minutes before my workout and another shake immediately following the workout. This works well for me, but the ideal timing for you may be different, depending on how fast your body digests the food, whether you are using a shake or whole food, and the reality of your life and schedule.

As a general rule, eat within two hours before your workout, and as soon as possible afterward.

"WHAT ABOUT WORKING OUT ON AN EMPTY STOMACH FIRST THING IN THE MORNING? I HEARD THAT THIS IS THE BEST WAY TO DO CARDIO FOR FAT BURNING."

If you work out on an empty stomach in the morning, you will burn more calories from fat initially, because you won't have glycogen in your system, which is the body's preferred fuel. However, the problem is that you risk also burning lean muscle. This is because your body is in a catabolic state in the morning because you have been fasting for typically eight hours or more. The consequence of losing lean muscle is that your metabolism slows down (remember from earlier chapters that lean muscle is the engine that drives your metabolism). So in the long term, skipping the preworkout shake or meal means that you will not be able to get as lean compared to having a small nutritious shake or meal before your cardio session.

You do not need a big meal with massive calories. I simply have a scoop of Juice Plus Complete, my favorite meal replacement shake. It contains only 130 calories. This small amount of calories will certainly not inhibit fat burning, but because the Complete shake is so nutrient dense it supplies my body with both the energy I need to get through my workout and the protein and nutrients I need to prevent muscle breakdown.

Another common fat-burning myth is that you should wait one to three hours after a cardio session to eat, in order to prolong the fat-burning effect. This practice sets you up to lose even more muscle and slow down your metabolism, especially if you follow this practice and do not eat before your workout.

While these strategies can be effective, I don't want to get too technical as that is not the goal of this book. I have found that most people don't need a better plan, a new diet, or a new supplement. They need to put focus, effort, and consistency, and a whole-hearted effort into the plan they already have.

In summary, my recommendation is to get some kind of nutrition before you work out in the morning. Also, make sure that you get plenty of pure water in your system before you work out.

"I HEARD THAT IT'S BEST NOT TO EAT AFTER 6:00 P.M. IF YOU WANT TO LOSE WEIGHT. IS THIS TRUE?"

I do not think that eating after 6:00 p.m. affects losing body fat, gaining lean muscle, or getting healthy. I know that many fitness professionals, nutritionists, and doctors will disagree with me, but my personal experience and experience with my clients indicates otherwise. I have personally achieved sub five percent body fat levels when I was getting ready for my natural bodybuilding contests, which is extremely lean, and I would always eat after 6 pm. In fact, sometimes I would get up in the middle of the night to get a meal in just so my muscles would not have to wait all night for a feeding. Yes, I know that I was crazy!

More important than the timing of your calories is the total number of calories you consume every day vs. the amount you burn. If you consume less than you burn, you will lose fat even if you eat after 6:00 p.m. (and may very well maintain more lean muscle).

The reason I believe people have success losing weight by not eating after 6:00 PM is that they are most likely eating less overall calories each day. Remember, any kind of restriction is going to naturally lower calories. This is analogous to a woman who, after cutting out all dairy, wheat, gluten, and processed carbs from her diet, is convinced that it was the carbs that was keeping her fat. This is not necessarily true. By removing all of these food items from her diet, she couldn't help but lose weight by significantly reducing her daily caloric intake.

Whether carbs, gluten, wheat, and dairy are bad for you and need to be removed from your diet is another topic and not within the scope of this book. I would, however, like to make just one brief comment on this topic. My opinion is that eating a balance of healthy foods in moderation, and focusing on getting lots of fresh fruits and vegetables in your diet is going to set you up for success. Too much of anything (except fruits and veggies) is not good, and a little bit of anything isn't going to hurt you too bad.

Therefore, not eating after 6:00 p.m. is not a big problem in terms of fitness and losing body fat. You should not, however, eat a very large meal right before bed (or any time of the day for that matter) if you're trying to lose body fat. There are cleansing and digestive benefits to having longer periods of fasting while you sleep, but again, it should not be an issue if you're not overeating or having large meals before bed.

"WHAT ABOUT ALCOHOL, RUSS? I LOVE TO HAVE MY RED WINE, AND I DON'T THINK I CAN GIVE IT UP."

Let's talk about the scientific facts first, and then talk reality. Alcohol contains about seven calories per gram, compared to four calories per gram of carbohydrates and protein and nine calories per gram of fat. The problem with alcohol calories is that our bodies cannot efficiently use them for energy. In fact, alcohol calories are nearly useless. Alcohol temporarily lowers metabolism and testosterone, which can quickly lead to increased fat storage. Not good so far, I know, but bear with me.

"BUT I HEARD RED WINE HAS RESVERATROL AND IS GOOD FOR MY HEART."

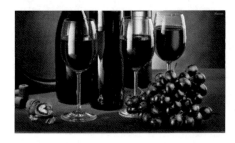

Yes, red wine does have antioxidants, and some studies indicate that a glass of red wine a day can provide cardiovascular benefits. However, other studies have questioned whether there are any health benefits from red wine. Moreover, there are other ways to get antioxidants besides wine.

Before you throw the book, curse me, and forget everything else I have taught you, let me make it perfectly clear that I enjoy a nice glass of red wine just as much as anyone else does. I have found that the key is to fit alcohol into your overall plan and enjoy it in moderation, just like anything else.

Technically, is it better not to drink alcohol at all? Yes, but it's also important that we enjoy life and take advantage of its pleasures. It is also technically healthier to never eat sugar, which would mean no cake, no ice cream, or pretty much any dessert! How boring would that be? While you can't overindulge *and* expect great health and a great body, it is possible to fit wine into an overall plan, reach your goals, and live a healthy and vibrant life.

So my suggestion is that if you choose to include alcohol in your life to enjoy it in moderation; stick to things like wine and beer and avoid hard liquor. Finally, limit yourself to one or two drinks in a sitting a few times a week. If you currently do not drink, I don't suggest that you start. This is one thing that you won't have to worry about!

"CAN I SAVE UP MY ONE OR TWO DRINKS A NIGHT AND HAVE THEM ALL IN ONE NIGHT?"

In terms of controlling your weight the answer is 'maybe' if you are in your teens or twenties, or if you have an exceptionally high metabolism. For most of us, however, the answer is 'No.' I've tried this and it doesn't work for several reasons. It's the same reason that you can't save up your calories and have them in one giant meal. Well, you can try, but you definitely will not get the same results as if you spread your calories out in the manner described in chapter 6.

Your body cannot process that many calories that fast, and this is going to slow down your metabolism. It is the same thing with alcohol, not to mention the other problems that may occur when you have many drinks at once. I don't think I need to explain this one!

In summary, if you are an elite athlete competing at a high level, I recommend refraining from alcohol altogether. Otherwise, it's OK to drink in moderation as long as you fit it into your overall nutrition and health plan.

NOTES/ACTION STEPS

CHAPTER 9:

WHICH SUPPLEMENTS DO I NEED TO TAKE?

A lthough this is the last chapter, that is often the first question that people ask me when they approach me in the gym or when they find out that I am a fitness professional.

Much to many a person's disappointment, who are wanting me to just tell them the "secret" pill, potion, or powder that will help them lose all the weight that they want without having to exercise or change their eating habits, and give them the energy they had in their teens with the sex drive to match (I am only *slightly* exaggerating), my initial response is to get them to take a step back and realize that the job of a supplement is just that; to *supplement* what they are not getting from their food.

It is important to understand that no amount of supplements will help you get measureable results unless you have a solid nutritional foundation first. This does not mean that your nutrition has to be perfect, as this is why supplements can be very useful. It is also important to understand that nutrition is just one piece of a bigger puzzle consisting of nutrition, sleep, strength training, and cardiovascular training. When all of these pieces are in place, certain supplements can give you an edge. Unfortunately, however, there is no magic pill.

I think the reason people look to supplements first is in hopes of finding a simple solution to all their problems. Although we know logically that this approach won't work, our hopes are raised by marketing from many supplement companies, and we end up wasting our hard-earned money on things that we don't need or, worse, are just plain worthless.

The only job of any supplement is to fill a gap between what we eat and what we need for optimal performance, energy, and health. When evaluating the need of nutritional products or supplements, I first start by seeing where the gaps are on a foundational basis. A gap exists where we need to be getting certain nutrients from our food but for whatever reason are not.

In actuality, we can get everything we need from food alone. The challenge is actually doing it with our busy lives. As I stated earlier, the average human needs to consume seven to thirteen servings of fruits and vegetables every day. That's a lot! And this is the recommendation for the average person and does not take into account high exercise or activity, which requires even more nutrients. Getting all the nutrients that we need can seem virtually impossible; this is where supplements can come into play.

When deciding on supplements, consider these three questions:

1) Does the product make sense?
2) Has the product been proven to do good things in the body by third-party clinical research?
3) Is the product safe and free of illegal or dangerous chemicals?

If a supplement passes these three tests I would say to give it a try and see how your body responds, as long as you remember rule number one about setting your foundation first.

"WHAT DO YOU THINK OF PROTEIN SHAKES AND BARS?"

After filling the gaps we have in terms of core vitamins, minerals, and antioxidants from natural food sources, the next level of supplementation consists of nutritional meal replacements, most often in the form of shakes and bars. Are they right for you? Again, it depends on what else you are you doing on an overall basis for your fitness and nutritional plan. No shake or bar alone can help you achieve great results.

It is important to note that all shakes and bars are not created equal. There are hundreds of different options out there; some are better than others. Unfortunately, many shakes and bars are nothing but glorified candy bars or milk shakes with a little bit of protein added in (which may or may not be quality protein), so make sure to read the ingredient labels.

You want to look for is something that is whole food based and natural. Just like reading food labels, if it lists things that sound like food, such as rolled oats, apples, raisins, and organic flax you are probably in good shape. If the label lists a bunch of things that sound like chemicals then you may want to consider if it is the type of "health food" you really want to put in your body!

If a supplement contains partially hydrogenated oil, run! Once you find options that meet the criteria above, it is important that you enjoy the taste enough to be able to use the products. The good news is that most shakes and bars these days taste much better than they did in the 1990s.

The third level of supplementation comprises products geared toward improving performance, burning fat, or building muscle. Examples that fall into this category are creatine, amino acids, electrolytes, and fat-burners. These can be effective in giving an elite athlete an extra edge over the competition. The majority of us do not need these products. I'm frustrated when I see so many people, especially young guys wanting to build muscle, immediately jump to using creatine, other muscle building products, or even anabolic steroids, while giving little consideration to what they eat.

Another classic example of looking for the miracle pill is the people who buy the latest and greatest fat-burner yet do not watch what they eat or even exercise regularly. Not only will supplements not help these people reach their goals, they can even be harmful if used improperly.

"I TAKE A MULTIVITAMIN EVERY DAY. WON'T THAT COVER ALL OF MY BASES?"

If you had asked me that prior to 2007, I would have given a very different answer than I give today. I unquestioningly took multivitamins my whole life, because that's what I was taught. Why shouldn't I? Everyone took vitamins, as we were told to by our parents and TV commercials, right? However, the truth of the matter is that all of the research that's been performed on multivitamins has shown no health benefits. That's right. In some cases, there has been evidence that using vitamins can actually cause harm to your body.

Without going into the research, which is outside the scope of this book, the reason isolated vitamins don't work is that our bodies are not vitamin deficient. They are whole food deficient. When we as humans start deciding which nutrients to put into vitamins it creates an unnatural imbalance in our bodies, especially if these are synthetic lab-made vitamins. We don't need mass amounts of individual vitamins, we need small amounts of all of the nutrients found in their natural state.

It amazes and frustrates me that, even though the research proves overwhelmingly that multivitamins provide little health benefit, people continue to spend billions of dollars on vitamins every year. Many people don't know the truth about multivitamins, while others know but don't know what to do. One of my missions is to spread the truth.

Don't believe me? Take a look at the American Heart Association and American Cancer Society websites. They have read the research and are now recommending diets rich in fruits and vegetables in place of multivitamin use.

So what's the answer? If not vitamins, as we had been taught from an early age, what should we take? The answer is that you should get nutrition from whole food sources, specifically from fruits and vegetables. Great! We have the answer. Fruits and vegetables are good for us. Big mystery solved. Knowing is only the beginning, however. Actually *doing it* is what counts!

It is quite another challenge to find all the fruits and vegetables, to be able to afford them, and to eat them all (or get your family to eat them all) before they spoil. Have you ever gone on a health kick and loaded up on fresh fruits and vegetables only to end up throwing more than half of them out at the end of the week? I have!

Two ways to make it easier to eat more fruits and vegetables are by making smoothies and juicing. These can be decent solutions, and I do like to make healthy and great-tasting smoothies. However, these two options still present a few challenges. They are time consuming, messy, and expensive. Juicing, especially, can be expensive, as it requires a tremendous amount of fruits and vegetables even for a small amount of juice. Can you say chop, slop, and mop?

One solution that I have found to be very effective, which I mentioned in chapter 7, is Juice Plus.

Juice plus takes twenty-eight fresh, raw fruits, vegetables, and berries that are grown in the field, picked at the peak of ripeness, dried at low temperatures, and put it into capsule or gummy form. Juice Plus provides a convenient, easy, and affordable way to fill the gap between the fruits and vegetables that we need every day and what we actually eat.

I have been taking Juice Plus since I found out about it in 2007, and recommend it to my clients as well. My clients and I continue to experience great results by adding Juice Plus to our diets. It is important to note that you still need to eat whole fruits and vegetables too. Juice Plus provides the necessary micronutrients (think antioxidants, vitamins, minerals, and other phytonutrients), but we still need the macronutrients and fiber that we can only get from whole fruits and vegetables.

Juice Plus has made it easier to get necessary macronutrients and fiber with whole-food-based replacement shakes and bars called Juice Plus Complete. My clients and I have experienced great success by following the Juice Plus Complete 60 Day Challenge to get big-time results fast in a healthy, maintainable fashion. I use Juice Plus Complete on a regular basis as a quick delicious source of whole food nutrition, and I use the 60 day challenge when I want to get in peak shape for a beach trip!

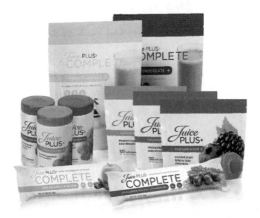

For more information on Juice Plus and to order products visit **www.russ.juiceplus.com**

These are the three products that I personally use every day and recommend. There are others, but these are the best that I have found.

I feel it necessary to include one last important note on children's vitamins. Even though this book is for women and men over thirty-five, I know that many of you have children, who are surely the most important part of your lives.

Many children's vitamins contain dangerous chemicals, such as red dyes, GMOs (genetically modified organisms), artificial sweeteners, and other chemicals that don't belong in children's bodies!

This is the actual warning label found on a popular children's vitamin:

"WARNING: Accidental overdose of iron-containing products is a leading cause of fatal poisoning in children under six. Keep this product out of reach of children. In case of accidental overdose, call a doctor or poison control center immediately."

I won't name names, but even a caveman could figure it out.

Think about that for a minute. Why in the world would we give something like this to our children? Our adult bodies don't know what to do with all these chemicals, and our children's bodies are even more sensitive and vulnerable than ours.

Our bodies, however, *do* know what to do with fruits and vegetables. For example, you will not find a warning label on the Juice Plus gummies. You won't even find a safety cap, because Juice Plus gummies are real food, and because they are safe.

Your children could literally eat the whole bag (a month's supply) and be fine. They may find themselves on the pot for a week, but that's a small price to pay!

The only warning I will give about the Juice Plus gummies is that they are ridiculously addictive. Please don't hold me accountable if you end up eating all of your children's gummies. I warned you!

I know this goes against everything you have heard your whole life about vitamins. You don't have to take my word for it. Do your own research and make your own decision regarding what is right for you and your family. As a fitness professional dedicated to helping as many people around the world live healthier lives, I feel it is my obligation to share what I know, even if it goes against common practice and beliefs.

Regardless of the supplementation plan or products you choose, remember to first establish a solid nutrition plan based on whole foods, then make sure that any supplements you decide to use are based on whole foods and have been proven by clinical research to be pure, safe, and effective.

NOTES/ACTION STEPS

BONUS CHAPTER: MOTIVATION, THE MENTAL EDGE, AND GETTING IT DONE!

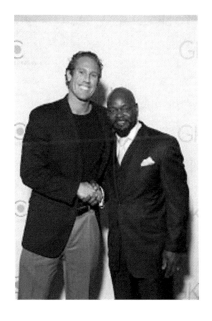

Russ and Emmitt Smith, NFL Hall of Fame running back.

Some of you will find this the most important chapter in the book.

Up to this point, I have given you all of the information that you need in order to successfully lose body fat safely, quickly, and permanently; to increase strength and energy; and to dramatically improve your health and vitality.

However, simply knowing the information is not enough. In order to win the prize, you must use what you have learned and *take action*. In this bonus chapter, I will share some of my best strategies for taking action and following through to help you obtain the body and health you desire.

I love finding and learning from other driven and successful people, from both an informational and motivational standpoint. I love the commercial where Emmitt Smith has just won the Super Bowl and he is bench-pressing. He says, "I know I can rest," and rests for about a second before busting out reps again.

Emmitt is an inspiration, and I was honored to meet him and learn some of his strategies for staying focused and motivated. I'm excited to share with you now the strategies I have learned and created over the years. Many of these strategies are much more mental than physical. The first of them is that...

YOU MUST HAVE A STRONG "WHY"

Before you attempt to make significant changes in your health, especially if your goal is to undergo a total physique transformation, you must have a strong motivation. Why do you want to do it? Lacking the "why," there is simply *no way* that you will stick to your plans and reach your goal. Your goal can be to win a physique transformation contest, to get ready for a beach trip, to make your ex's head spin when you see him or her at your reunion, or to be able to keep up with your kids while doing the things you once enjoyed but are now too tired to do. It does not matter what that reason is, only that it is important to *you*. Make sure that you take the time to ask yourself exactly why you are doing this and remind yourself of that reason throughout your journey.

MOTIVATION

Motivation and your "why" work together synergistically. It is great to have a "why," but it is important to generate the motivation to follow through with what you know you *need* to be doing but may not *feel* like doing. Motivation is the reason that we get out of bed in the morning and start our day. It is what drives us to get to the gym and work harder than we did the day before. Motivation is the reason that great ideas turn into great accomplishments. Motivation is what drives us to get things done!

Motivation exists in many different forms and can come from external sources or can be self-generated. Think about what motivates you to get to work in the morning. For many of us, the motivation is survival. We need to work in order to make money, so that we can survive. Others are motivated to get to work because they truly love their jobs and can't wait to improve their business or make a difference in the lives of others. For others, the motivation is knowing that if they don't get to work on time, they will be out of a job!

How can we use motivation to help us in our efforts to transform our physique and health? Any way you can and as much as you can! If you need to boost your motivation to get to the gym or to work out hard, look at photos of exemplary physiques you admire or watch a fitness video

featuring someone you admire. Sometimes seeing others succeed through hard work (especially at the same thing you
are doing) can be extremely motivating. You can also use the
opposite tack, to look at pictures of yourself in which you
are out of shape. This can quickly remind you that you have
changed your workout and eating habits and that you will
never go back to your old self again!

SURROUND YOURSELF WITH A POSITIVE SUPPORT SYSTEM

It has been said time and again that we are the sum of the five
people we spend the most time with. Another way to say this
is that the best way to achieve greatness is to surround yourself
with people who have already achieved it. Having role models
and copying their strategies is an extremely effective way to
achieve success in anything you do in life, including making
a dramatic change in your physique, health, and fitness. Find
people who have achieved what you want to achieve. Also,
find out what they do to achieve success. You can apply the
same proven strategies to help you achieve similar, or even
better, results.

Try to associate yourself with positive people who have
goals and interests similar to your own. Having a close net-
work of such people can have a huge impact on your motivation and ability to follow through with your program.
Reading motivational books and articles is a great strategy
as well. It does not even have to have anything to do with
fitness or working out. It is easy to become inspired by others who have passionately and persistently achieved greatness, no matter what their endeavor.

NEVER LISTEN TO THE OPINIONS OF NEGATIVE PEOPLE!

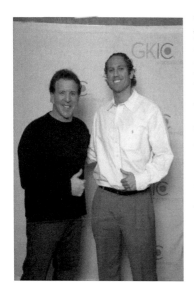

Jake Steinfeld, best known for Body By Jake, is a perfect example of someone who did not listen to naysayers. Others repeatedly told him that he couldn't be successful, but he didn't listen. Jake went on to build an empire and is by far the wealthiest personal trainer in the world, with a net worth of over $600 million.

He is a brilliant businessman, a genuine person, a family man, and a great role model, if you ask me.

Unfortunately, there are people who like to put others down and tell them that they cannot succeed. Even though such people may discourage you and cause you to question what you are doing, you must fight to not let that happen. Often, the real reason that such people may disparage you has nothing to do with you at all. It's about satisfying their own insecurities and proving to themselves that their way of life is right and that yours must be wrong. They are trying to build themselves up by tearing you down. Don't listen to them for even a second!

It can be human nature to try to prevent others from changing for the better, especially if they are not willing to change themselves, because they feel like they will get left behind.

Instead of arguing with bitter people who will not change their minds, use their negative attitudes to fuel your motivation even more. If something makes you angry, take it out on the weights. I have had some of my best workouts after becoming angry. Also, remember that these naysayers have nothing invested in your life and your decisions. You are the one making the investment in yourself, so believe in yourself, and don't worry about what others think.

HAVE A DEADLINE

In order to achieve measureable results in a reasonable period of time, you *must* have a clear deadline. Trust me on this! You don't necessarily have to compete in a physique competition (although I think this can be an excellent motivation), but lacking a clear deadline makes it way too easy to get off track. Without a deadline, it becomes much easier to reach for the piece of pizza or cheesecake at dinner. Why not? You can finish your transformation goal a little later than planned. That's not to say that you can't incorporate pizza or cheesecake into your plan (we discussed how to do that in chapter 6), but if you can always put off your task until tomorrow, temporary pleasure will triumph over consistently making the best choices. A firm deadline creates focus and purpose. Focus and purpose produce results!

PLANNING AND PREPARATION

The important role of planning and preparation in a successful physique transformation, or any health program, cannot be underestimated. Both physical and mental preparation are equally important. While you may find your challenges unique, I guarantee that everyone has to deal with similar challenges that life presents—whether a stressful job, kids, travel, and more.

However, it is still possible to stay on track with your training and nutrition plan if you prepare and plan properly. This is a lesson I learned during my participation in the AST World Championships, a physique transformation competition. Every weekend, I went to the grocery store to buy all the food I would need for the upcoming week. I then cooked up enough food to last a few days, or for the whole week if I was going to be traveling out of town that week. I traveled about 30 percent of the time during the AST World Championships and often worked long hours. But with planning and preparation, I was able to stay on track and not miss a beat. Without proper planning and preparation, any small curve ball can throw off all the positive momentum you have built.

If you are always prepared, you control your circumstances; they do not control you. Does it take some time and thought? Sure, but the prize of looking and feeling awesome is so worth it! Additionally, you will save the time and energy involved in deciding where to go for lunch and in driving there and back. Cooking your own healthy food can even help you save a lot of money that you would have otherwise spent eating out!

KEEP A TRAINING AND NUTRITION JOURNAL

A training and nutrition journal is a very valuable tool in any health and fitness program. It allows you to accurately track your progress, but more importantly, it holds you accountable for everything you do or don't do. If you want to truly make an outstanding physique transformation, keeping a training journal is *absolutely essential.* If you lack the discipline to keep track of your workouts and nutrition, you can forget about making the kind of transformation that will amaze friends and family. Have your fitness coach review your training journal at least weekly. This will help keep you on track; who wants their fitness coach to read that they are not doing what they know they should be doing?

Once you get the hang of keeping a journal, it actually becomes quite enjoyable. You don't have to stick strictly to sets, reps, and calories. Write about how you felt that day or about a particular challenge you overcame. A training journal kept during a physique transformation can serve as an excellent resource in future fitness endeavors and can also motivate others to make their own transformation.

If you follow only one nutritional strategy from this book, it should be to *write down* everything you eat each day, or instead, to use one of the many apps on your phone that allow you to track your daily food intake. The act of writing it down makes you more aware of what you eat. Sometimes I use the following trick with new clients: I tell them that they can eat anything they like for the first month. The only catch is that they must write down everything they eat, no matter what. In every single case, the client naturally began making better choices simply as a result of writing it down and being aware of what they were eating.

BE IN CONTROL OF THE SITUATION AND NOT THE OTHER WAY AROUND

As you start your fitness program, rest assured that you will come across obstacles that make it difficult to stick to your plan. You always have choices. Although they will not always be easy, they are yours to make. Take responsibility for every action you take, and always be in control of your situation. This ties in with planning and preparation, as well as having a burning desire to succeed. If you want it badly enough, prove it, and do what you set out to do in the first place. If you do make a poor decision, take responsibility for it, and get right back on your plan. The emotional pain you go through when straying from your plan will help prevent recurrence in the future.

It is important to know yourself and your patterns. If you can truly limit yourself to one small serving of "fun" food, such as a slice of pizza or a cookie, that is fine and will not mess up your progress. However, if you are like me and know that the first piece of pizza or cookie will lead to all your will power going out the window and turn into a chow-down session, it is best to refrain altogether.

DON'T MAKE EXCUSES

One of my business partners says, "You can make money, or you can make excuses, but you can't make both." The same can be said about making progress with your health and fitness goals. Don't fall into the habit of making poor choices that you justify with excuses. While this may temporarily make you feel better, it will only cause emotional pain and failure in the long run. There will *always* be someone who is better, stronger, faster, leaner, wealthier, or smarter. Some people just plain have it easier than you do.

Don't waste your time and energy focusing on such inequalities. First of all, you usually have no idea what those people have gone through to achieve the apparent *easy* life they have. Even if they have had it easier, what good will it do you to blame your lack of good fortune and make excuses for your shortcomings? None! Concentrate all your physical, mental, and emotional effort into being the best *you* that you can be. If you do that, you will be successful no matter what. If you continue to make excuses, you won't. Gratitude is one of the best ways to bring more good things into your life, and the most positive and useful emotion that exists.

The first thing I do when I wake up is to state out loud three things I am grateful for in my life. Often times, I will state more than three things, but that is the starting point. I really attempt to not only say what I am grateful for but focus on it and "feel" it. I started this habit years ago and it really does make a positive difference in your day.

I repeat the process in the evenings right before I go to sleep. Try it out and I think you will be happy with the results. Fear is the emotion that most often holds us back from accomplishing our dreams. One of my mentors taught me that it is impossible to be grateful and fearful at the same time. Get grateful and eliminate fear from your life!

TREAT EACH WORKOUT AS IF IT WERE AN APPOINTMENT WITH YOUR BOSS

How many workouts have you blown off in the past year? How about meetings with your boss? I'm guessing that the first number is much higher, but it shouldn't be. Of course, being responsible and accountable to the person who pays you every two weeks is extremely important, but so is your commitment to your health and fitness. Health and fitness are some of the most neglected areas in our lives. This is not only sad; it's downright scary. The money spent on doctors and hospital bills, the lost time at work, and heartache that diseases cause families are simply staggering. Regular exercise and eating healthy food have each been proven to *significantly* reduce the likelihood of developing heart disease, diabetes, numerous types of cancer, and many other illnesses. The synergistic benefits of exercise and good nutrition together are very powerful. Knowing this information, how can taking care of yourself not be a priority?

I can't think of anything more important, in order to live a long and happy life, than taking care of your health and your body. Having a killer body is just a nice side effect. Treat yourself with respect, and don't miss your workout appointments. Schedule your workouts on your calendar, and make them happen!

USE THE POWER OF MUSIC TO FUEL YOUR WORKOUTS

There is just something about music and the energy it provides to fuel your workouts. Studies have proven this theory. I don't know exactly how this works, but I do know that my motivation and energy seem to skyrocket when my favorite music is blasting! An MP3 player, such as the iPod, is one of the best investments you can make to create more enjoyable workouts. You can even listen to audio books during cardio, like I do. A strategy I have recently adopted is to listen to a business or educational book the first half of my cardio session, and then crank out some tunes for the second half of my cardio workout.

I prefer hard rock when I am lifting weights. It really gets my blood pumping and motivation high! When I am performing cardio I am all about audio books. I have always loved to read and learn, but found it difficult to make the time for reading. Audio books are the perfect answer as you can listen to them while you are working out or driving in your car so it requires no extra time. I try to find efficiencies wherever I can in life and audio books have been a big one for me.

KEEP YOUR EYE ON THE PRIZE

Completing a fitness and nutrition plan is one of the most rewarding physical, mental, and emotional experiences you can undergo. However, we all know that nothing worth having comes without a "price tag." At times, you will undoubtedly feel tired, hungry, frustrated, and ready to give up. You will ask yourself why you are putting yourself through this ordeal while your friends are out enjoying themselves, eating pizza, and drinking beer. These are the times you have to remind yourself of your *why* (remember my first tip?). Focus is a special thing. If you remain focused on your goal and stay motivated, nothing can stop you. Keep your eye on the prize; it will be yours in the end. If you can stay really focused for a few months, you can make dramatic progress. Once you reach your ideal body shape and health, continue to follow the principles that got you there in the first place. You can also learn how to balance your new healthy lifestyle with a normal lifestyle.

CONCLUSION AND THE
ULTIMATE FAT FLUSH PROGRAM

We have discussed how to lose weight safely, quickly, and permanently; the right kind of weight to lose for permanent weight loss; and the planning and strategies necessary to accomplish your goals. We talked about the best time to work out; various types of workout programs, as well as their pros and cons; and dispelled the myth that lifting weights will make you big and bulky.

Next, we talked about nutrition and its important role in achieving a lean and healthy physique, as well as in creating abundant energy and long-term health. We talked about meal timing, macronutrients, micronutrients, and the importance of getting lots of fruits and vegetables into your daily diet. We also discussed the confusing array of diets out there, as well as the type of supplementation that can help us reach our goals, and what is nothing more than a waste of money.

Lastly, we talked about *implementation*: taking action and getting it done! I shared some specific strategies that have helped both me and my clients achieve success.

You are now armed with more than enough information to create the physique and health of your dreams. Now that you know how to sift through the mass of confusing and conflicting information on working out and eating—in a way that helps you permanently lose weight and increase your energy—I challenge you to take action on the information you have learned.

It has been said that knowledge is power. In reality, knowledge is power only when applied. Without action, nothing will change!

I absolutely love what I do and wish that I could work individually with everyone who wants more out of health and life. While that is impossible, I feel like through this book hopefully you and I have made a connection and that I have made a positive influence in your life, even if it is small. If it is big then that is even better!

It has been an honor to spend this short time with you, and I truly wish that you have the health, energy, and body that you desire!

If you would like to continue our relationship and let me help you on this journey, call me at (678) 867–0101 or go to www.UltimateFatFlush.com to take advantage of a special program I have put together designed to help you lose fat and increase energy quickly, safely, and permanently—all at a very special price.

My sincere wish for you is that you use the information in this book, and commit to looking and feeling your best ever and becoming your *BEST YOU NOW*!

Thank you, and remember that you can do anything that you set your mind to!

To Your Extraordinary Health!

-Russ